CALORIE
COUNTER

MAGGIE PANNELL

SUNBURST BOOKS

This edition first published in 1995 by
Sunburst Books,
Deacon House,
65 Old Church Street,
London SW3 5BS.

© Sunburst Books 1995

ISBN 1 85778 152 X

Printed and bound in China

ACKNOWLEDGEMENT
The publishers would like to thank the Royal Society of
Chemistry for their co-operation during the production of
this book.

PUBLISHER'S NOTE
Neither the publisher nor the author takes any
responsibility for the implementation of any
recommendations, ideas or techniques expressed
and described in this book. Any use to which the
recommendations, ideas and techniques are put is at
the reader's sole discretion and risk.

CONTENTS

INTRODUCTION

What Are Calories?

All food provides energy in the form of fats, proteins and carbohydrates, and it's measured in calories (or joules, under the metric system). We need this energy as a 'fuel' for all the chemical reactions which take place in the body, even when we are asleep. Everything we do requires energy, from simply breathing and keeping warm to all kinds of physical activity. However, if we eat food that is surplus to our requirements, this excess energy is not 'burned' by the body but instead is stored as fat.

What Are Your Calorie Needs?

Different people require different amounts of energy, depending on their height, build, sex, age, level of activity and individual metabolism. Metabolism is a global word covering all those chemical changes that go on in the body, and metabolic rate is the speed at which they occur or the rate at which food is burned in order to produce energy.

Generally men have a higher metabolic rate than women because men have much more body muscle, which is an active energy-burning tissue. The female body is more padded with relatively inactive fat. As we grow older, muscles tend to waste away as we slow down and generally become less physically active. This lowers the metabolic rate and therefore reduces our calorie requirement, so older people find they do not need to eat as much as they used to.

Your level of activity is a significant factor influencing what your calorie intake should be. Someone who has a very physically demanding job, such as a builder or gardener, obviously needs more energy than someone who's sitting behind a desk for most of the day. Regrettably, recommended figures for calorie intake are lower than they used to be as a result of modern life styles, with many more people in sedentary jobs, using labour-saving devices and travelling by car and other forms of transport.

> **The estimated average requirement for women aged 19-50 years is 1960 Calories per day. The estimated average requirement for men of the same age is 2550 Calories per day. (1 Calorie=1 Kilocalorie=1000 calories.)**

It's only as a result of the increasing incidence of diet-related diseases in the Western world that we are now becoming more health conscious and are paying more attention to the link between diet, exercise, lifestyle and health. However, although we know that height, sex, age and level of activity all influence metabolic rate, individuals still vary enormously.

Some people just seem to be very efficient at burning calories and appear to be able to eat as much of whatever they like. Others, rather unfairly, only have to look at a bar of chocolate and the weight seems to pile on. Certainly you can increase your metabolic rate by taking more exercise, but maintaining a desirable body weight is largely a matter of knowing how many calories you can eat without putting on weight.

The Calorie Value of Food

All foods have a calorie value, which depends on the nutrient content of the food. Fats provide twice as many calories as carbohydrates and proteins, so foods that are high in fat, such as cream, hard cheese, chocolate, pastries, but-terand so on have a high calorie value. It's also been suggested that fat causes more weight gain than the same amount of calories from other foods. Vitamins and minerals are also nutrients but do not provide energy or, therefore, calories. Foods that have a high water content, such as salad vegetables, are low in calories because there are no calories in water. There is also a component in foods of vegetable origin, including cereals, pulses, fruit, vegetables and nuts, called dietary fibre, or non-starch polysaccharides (NSP). Animal products do not contain fibre. The fibre component of a food has no calorie value because it is not digested. Fibre-rich foods not only encourage a healthy digestion, but are of great benefit to slimmers because they take longer to chew and, being comparatively bulky, give a feeling of fullness.

The healthiest way to eat is to choose a variety of foods that are nutritious without giving us more calories than we need. Most foods are made up of a combination of nutrients. Bread, for example, provides carbohydrate and protein (both of which provide energy or calories), as well as calcium, iron and B vitamins. Protein also provides material for growth, tissue repair and is good for bone development. There's no need to eat any one food in particular, because with a varied diet you will certainly get all the nutrients you need from various different sources, which together will provide sufficient energy. Don't cut out starchy carbohydrates such as rice, pasta, bread and potatoes. They are not in themselves fattening when eaten in moderate quantities, but are good, sustaining fillers.

Wholegrain varieties are a particularly good source of fibre, vitamins and minerals. It's the fats eaten with these foods that can make them high in calories.

Some foods, however, are less nourishing than others. They provide so-called 'empty calories' because there's little else in them other than energy value. Confectionery, biscuits, cakes, and many snack foods fall into this category. They have a high sugar and/or fat content and provide a lot of unnecessary calories. Far better to have a piece of fruit as a snack, which with just 40 Calories or so provides both valuable fibre and vitamins. Sweet foods, however, have a very high calorie value as well as being bad for the teeth. The sugar quickly enters the blood stream and gives you an immediate 'lift'. However, the blood sugar level rapidly drops again, leaving you feeling tired and lethargic, so the tendency is to reach for something else to eat. In essence, the sweet snack has not been sustaining, yet you've still taken in all those calories – 200 Calories or more – for a bar of chocolate.

Consequences of Over-eating

You may not think you're eating a lot, but if you add up all the snacks between meals, eating the children's leftovers, nibbling while cooking and so on, they all add to your daily calorie intake. So don't deceive yourself. Keep a food diary and write down everything you have eaten, with its calorie value. It's not so much the quantity you eat, but the choice of food that matters. If your diet includes a lot of biscuits, cakes, chocolate, crisps, fried food, alcoholic and sugary drinks, the calories quickly mount up and you can soon become overweight.

Excess weight means the heart has to pump much harder and this puts up blood pressure, which in time causes damage to the blood vessels and interferes with blood flow to vital organs. If not detected, kidney failure, heart disease and strokes can follow. If overweight, you're more likely to suffer from circulatory and respiratory problems, late onset diabetes and arthritis. A high fat diet is also known to be a contributing factor in causing heart disease.

Losing Weight

If you're overweight, you need to reduce your calorie intake and step up your exercise level. Then, your body will automatically draw on fat reserves for energy and you'll start to lose weight. You don't have to give up all your favourite foods, just eat sensibly.

Body fat weighing 454 g/1lb is equivalent to 3500 Calories, so to lose just 454g/1lb you need to restrict your intake by 3500 Calories. Given that the average woman, with moderate activity, uses approximately 2000 Calories a day to maintain weight, following a 1000-Calorie-a-day diet, you stand to lose 908g/2lb in 7 days, or 1 week. This sounds slow, but steady weight loss is healthier and more likely to stay off. It also gives your metabolism, skin and muscles time to adjust to your new shape and size.

Never try to follow a very low calorie diet (under 600 Calories a day) for any length of time. Not only is this unhealthy – it can cause muscle wastage and damage to organs such as the liver – but such diets are doomed to fail because they provide so very little food. You will feel tired, hungry and depressed, which leads to cheating. You may also suffer side effects, such as giddiness, headaches, nausea, irregular periods and cramps. Very low calorie diets also tend to slow down your metabolism, so on returning to an increased calorie intake, weight goes back on more easily.

Meal replacements, which depend on specially formulated milk shakes and biscuits, are also not to be recommended for long term dieting. Certainly they can be useful for the occasional quick 'meal' and some people claim to have great success using them, but they don't retrain your eating habits. It's then all too easy to slip back into old habits after dieting, and the weight goes back on.

The Healthy Way to Diet

The main reason why so many diets fail is that they are inflexible: choice of foods is severely restricted; they can be unappetising; and favourite foods are forbidden. After all, why do we eat? Apart from nourishing the body for growth, repair and energy, we eat for pleasure. If that enjoyment is removed, then it is hardly surprising that the regime becomes impossible to stick to. To be successful, a diet should include a wide variety of foods. The following should be used as guidelines to a healthier diet.

* Select wholefoods, plenty of fresh fruit and vegetables, lean meat, skinned poultry and fish, wholewheat cereals and pulses and low-fat dairy produce. Choose 'healthy' foods and you'll find you can eat much more than you could by snacking on high-fat and high-sugar convenience foods.

* Eating a wholefood diet will also increase your intake of fibre, from wholegrain cereals, pulses, nuts, fresh and dried fruits, root and

leafy vegetables. High-fibre foods are very filling so your appetite is satisfied at meal times and the temptation to nibble in between meals shouldn't arise.

* Aim to have regular meals. This helps keep your metabolism ticking over and reduces the temptation to snack indiscriminately.

* Eating little and often is fine, if it suits your lifestyle better, provided the light meals/snacks you choose are healthy ones: for example, a wholemeal sandwich, a salad or a yogurt with fruit.

* When shopping, look for all the reduced-fat and lower-sugar alternatives.

* Eat less red meat and more fish, poultry and pulses. This will help you to reduce your overall fat intake and therefore calorie intake. (*See* the section 'How to reduce calories in cooking' on page 19.)

* Eat a good variety of fruit and vegetables (aim for 5 servings a day), and choose fresh fruit or raw vegetables as a snack between meals rather than reaching for a chocolate biscuit or a bag of crisps.

APPLE - **40 Calories**
1 CHOCOLATE BISCUIT - **85 Calories**
BAG OF CRISPS - **135 Calories**

* Restrict all high fat and sugary foods. Reserve these for occasional treats.

* Include plenty of fluids in your diet – at least 6-8 drinks a day – but remember that calories in drinks can add up. For example, 6 cups of tea/coffee a day with whole milk would add up to about 340 Calories, whereas if they were made with skimmed milk they would add up to about 175 Calories, a saving of 165 Calories. Similarly, watch your alcohol intake, use low-calorie mixers and drink as much water as possible.

The Importance of Exercise

The best way to lose weight is not only to eat healthily but also to increase the amount of physical exercise while you are slimming. This means that you can allow yourself a little more food and still lose weight. You'll also look fitter as the exercise helps tone up slack muscles, improves posture and helps you feel more vital and alert.

<u>KEY</u>

UNDERWEIGHT
You are not eating enough and could do
with gaining a little weight.

OK
This is the desirable weight range for
your health.

OVERWEIGHT
Unlikely to have a serious effect on your
health, but don't put on further weight.
Choose your food more carefully.

FAT
Your health could suffer if you don't lose
weight.

VERY FAT
This is severe and strict dieting and
exercise is urgently necessary. Your
health may already be suffering.

HEIGHT / WEIGHT CHART

Are you the right weight for your height?
The chart indicates the weight category into which you fall –
normal, fat, underweight and so on.

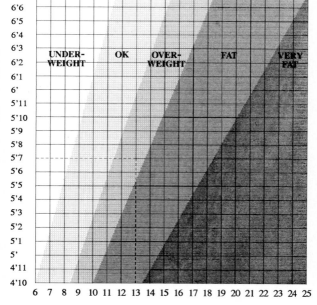

Your height in feet and inches (1 foot = approx 0.3 metres)

Your weight in stones (1 pound = approx 0.45 kilograms)

Chart from *Treat Obesity Seriously*, J S Garrow,
Churchill Livingstone Edinburgh 1981

There's no need to take up an energetic sport. In fact you shouldn't if you're not used to vigorous exercise. Take it at your own pace and don't over-exert yourself. You can exercise simply by walking or cycling rather than using the car for short trips, going for an evening swim rather than sitting in front of the television, climbing the stars rather than taking the lift. Exercise should be enjoyed. Regular gentle exercise is better than occasional bursts.

The chart below gives some examples of the calories you can use up by exercising.

LEVEL OF ACTIVITY	CALORIES USED PER HALF HOUR	EXERCISE
LIGHT	100	walking housework light gardening
MODERATE	200	cycling energetic dancing brisk walking, digging, gentle swimming
STRENUOUS	300	keep fit jogging tennis football fast swimming

Reducing Calories in Cooking

Around 40 per cent of the calories we eat come from fats. Experts recommend that we should cut that figure down to between 30-35 per cent, which means cutting fat intake, particularly saturated fats, by a quarter. Saturated fats are hard fats, such as those used in cakes, biscuits, chocolate, pastries and savoury snacks as well as dairy products such as butter, cream, cheese and red meat. Eating less fat can be done quite easily by shopping wisely and by making some simple cooking adjustments.

Red meat, even when lean, is quite high in fat, so choose more fish and poultry (skinned) instead and allow smaller portions of meat per person. Quantities can be bulked up in recipes with pulses, such as in chilli con carne, or with larger servings of vegetables or salad.

Choose leaner cuts of meat. Many animals are now actually bred to be leaner and consequently there is a far greater selection of lean cuts. Trim excess fat off meat and remove skin from poultry before cooking.

Do not add extra fat to meat when browning in a frying pan. If you use a non-stick pan, even with trimmed lean meat, there's usually sufficient hidden fat in the lean tissue to brown the meat without it sticking. Poultry may need a little oil but any excess should be drained off.

Always grill, oven bake or microwave whenever possible, rather than fry. When it is necessary to fry use a non-stick pan, strain off excess fat after frying and drain food on a piece of absorbent kitchen paper.

Roast meat on a rack so the fat drains through underneath.

Don't pre-cook vegetables in oil for casseroles, soups and so on, but incorporate them raw into the sauce.

Use low-fat natural (plain) yoghurt in place of cream. If it's to be heated, stabilise the yoghurt first by blending a little cornflour into it (one tsp cornflour to 150ml / ¼ pint yoghurt).

Cut bread and chips thicker so that there's less surface area for fat to be absorbed. It's better to have one thick slice of bread, thinly spread with butter or an alternative, than two thin slices both spread with fat.

100g/4 oz of thick-cut chips have about 190 Calories compared to 280 Calories for thin-cut French fries. Chips and all fried foods generally are high in calories. Choose a baked jacket potato or new boiled, rather than fried.

Hard cheese is very high in fat and calories. Try half-fat varieties or use less of a stronger flavoured hard cheese, such as parmesan. Try curd cheese instead of cream cheese.

Substitute semi-skimmed or skimmed milk in place of whole milk.

Eating Out
Choose plain grilled, baked or steamed dishes rather than anything that has been fried, prepared in breadcrumbs, batter or pastry.

Choose salads with light dressings and steamed and stir-fried vegetables, not those in sauces.

If you would like a dessert choose fresh fruit salad, crème caramel or sorbet.

Watch the cheese board. See the Calorie Counter for lower calorie choices; do not put butter on the biscuits or bread roll.

Have mineral water as well as wine to reduce the amount of alcohol you drink.

Using the Calorie Counter

The great thing about counting calories is that you can choose what you want to eat to suit your own lifestyle and individual likes and dislikes. Nothing need be banned, just limited to special occasions or treats.

However, with calorie counting you must be strict with yourself. You must, initially at least, weigh yourself correctly and write down absolutely everything you eat, adding up your total for each day and keeping within your allowance. Making a wrong guess about a high calorie food such as a piece of cheese could cost you quite heavily in the calorie stakes: there are 120 Calories in 28g /1oz of Cheddar cheese but 240 Calories in 56g /2oz. Once you've become familiar with portion sizes, you can make judgements based on sound experience.

It may seem a little boring at first but you'll soon learn calorie values for common foods without having to look them up, and will be able to do calculations quite quickly in your head. Moreover, dieting is largely a matter of common sense. Choose a healthy diet, as described, and the calories will largely take care of themselves.

Determine your calorie allowance for the whole week to allow yourself some flexibility. It's your

Food Groups	Amount	Calories	Amount	Calories
Apples, eating	100 g	42	1 oz	12
avg whole fruit	113 g	48	4 oz	48
cooking	100 g	26	1 oz	7
avg whole fruit	227 g	56	8 oz	56
apple sauce, sweetened	227 tbsp	20		
apple sauce, unsweetened	1 tbsp	10		
Apricots, fresh	100 g	29	1 oz	8
avg whole fruit	28 g	8	1 oz	8
dried (without stones)	100 g	158	1 oz	44
per dried fruit		10		

overall eating pattern that counts, not individual
days. So if you know that you are going out for a
meal, watch calories very strictly before and you
can indulge yourself on the special occasion.

The calories in the Calorie Counter (*see* the
example, above) have been given both per 100g
and per 1oz of food, so be sure to read the correct
figure. There are also spoon measurements where
it is considered to be more helpful, and average
portion sizes and calories per individual item

where appropriate – but remember, these can only be average figures.

In ready-prepared meals there is a great deal of variation between different recipes, and the manufacturers' portion sizes vary from being somewhat mean to quite generous. The calories quoted here for ready-prepared dishes have been based on average values and should be used as a guide only; always check the nutrition panels on the side of packets for the actual calorie count.

Calorie counting allows you plenty of variety and freedom of choice, which are essential if you're going to be successful.

Once you've reached your target weight, you can increase your calorie intake to a level at which you can maintain your weight.

But remember, in order to maintain your weight at its new level, you should stick to the healthy food choices you've learned while dieting, and also keep up the exercise. If you follow this advice then weight watching should never be a problem again.

CALORIFIC VALUES
OF FOOD

BREAD AND STAPLE CEREALS

Food Groups	Amount	Calories	Amount	Calories
BREADS				
Wholemeal/brown	100g	215	1 oz	60
	1 thick slice	90		
White bread	100 g	235	1 oz	66
	1 thick slice	100		
High fibre white	100 g	227	1 oz	64
	1 thick slice	96		
French stick	100 g	270	1 oz	76
1 slice	50 g	135	1¾ oz	135
Granary	100 g	235	1 oz	66
	1 thick slice	100		
Breadcrumbs, fresh	1 tbsp	20		
dried	1 tbsp	30		
Bread rolls				
soft white	100 g	268	1 oz	75
per item,	60 g	156		

FOOD GROUPS	AMOUNT	CALORIES	AMOUNT	CALORIES
wholemeal	100 g	241	1 oz	67
per item,	60g	144		
small bridge roll	15 g	35	½ oz	35
Hamburger bap	per item	130		
Bagel, plain	per item	170		
cinnamon & raisin	per item	225		
Brioche	100 g	352	1 oz	98
Chollah	100	265	1 oz	74
Chappati	per item	140		
Croissant, avg	56 g	190	2 oz	190
Grissini	per item	20		
Nann bread, plain, avg	per item	340	135 g	340
flavoured,	per item	365		
peshwari, fruited	per item	515		
Oat cake	per item	60		
Paratha	per item	450		
Pitta bread, white	100 g	260	1 oz	73

Food Groups	Amount	Calories	Amount	Calories
Pitta bread (cont)				
per item,	70g	185		
wholemeal	100 g	235	1 oz	66
per item,	70g	165		
mini	per item	90		
party-size	per item	45		
Puppodum	per item	52		
Pumpernickel/rye bread	100 g	219	1 oz	61
per slice	109	50		
Pasta - dry white, raw	100 g	342	1 oz	96
Macaroni white, raw	1 US cup	384	4 oz	384
white (cooked)	100 g	104	1 oz	30
avg portion (starter) dry	56 g	192	2 oz	192
avg portion (main) dry	85 g	290	3 oz	290
wholewheat, raw	100 g	325	1 oz	90
Macaroni, wholewheat raw	1 US cup	360	4 oz	360
wholewheat, cooked	100 g	113	1 oz	32

Food Groups	Amount	Calories	Amount	Calories
Pasta, fresh, avg, cooked	100 g	163	1 oz	46
avg portion (main)				
tagliatelle, cooked		317		
avg portion, (main)				
stuffed pasta;				
eg ravioli, cooked		360		
Egg noodles, boiled	100 g	62	1 oz	17
Rice, brown, raw	100 g	357	1 oz	100
	1 US cup	650	6½ oz	650
cooked	100 g	140	1 oz	40
	50 g (dry wt)	178		
Rice, white, raw	100 g	383	1 oz	107
	1 US cup	695	6½ oz	695
cooked	100 g	138	1 oz	39
avg portion (dry wt)	50 g	165		
Basmati, cooked	100 g	121	1 oz	34
avg portion	50 g (dry wt)	165		

Food Groups	Amount	Calories	Amount	Calories
pilau, cooked	100 g	193	1 oz	54
pudding rice, cooked	100 g	102	1 oz	29
avg portion	140 g	134	4½ oz	134
risotto, cooked with oil				
butter + stock	100g	224	1oz	63
avg portion	50 g (dry wt)	209		
savoury, raw	100 g	415	1 oz	116
cooked	100 g	142	1 oz	40
wild rice, raw	100 g	375	1 oz	105
	1 US cup	682	6½ oz	682
cooked	100 g	175	1 oz	49
Bran, wheat	100g	206	1 oz	58
	1 US cup	232	4 oz	232
	1 tbsp	17		
Bulgar wheat, cooked	100 g	103	1 oz	29
	1 tbsp	38		
Couscous, raw	100 g	375	1 oz	105

FOOD GROUPS	AMOUNT	CALORIES	AMOUNT	CALORIES
couscous, cooked	100 g	235	1 oz	66
avg serving	75g	177		
Oats, raw	100 g	375	1 oz	105
	1 US cup	320	3 oz	320
Pearl barley, raw	100 g	364	1 oz	102
	1 US cup	714	7 oz	714
cooked	100 g	122	1 oz	34
Cornflour/custard powder	100g	354	1 oz	99
cornstarch	1 tbsp	64		
Flour, white	100 g	340	1 oz	95
	1 US cup	380	4 oz	380
wholemeal	100g	310	1 oz	87
wholemeal	1 US cup	348	4 oz	348
white/wholemeal	1 tbsp	35		
Wheatgerm	100 g	357	1 oz	100
	1 tbsp	18		
Shortcrust pastry, raw	100 g	450	1 oz	126

Food Groups	Amount	Calories	Amount	Calories
shortcrust pastry, cooked	100 g	520	1 oz	145
Puff pastry, raw	100 g	410	1 oz	115
cooked	100 g	540	1 oz	152
Filo pastry, raw	100 g	315	1 oz	88
cooked	100 g	395	1 oz	110

BREAKFAST CEREALS

Food Groups	Amount	Calories	Amount	Calories
All Bran	100 g	260	1 oz	73
avg portion	56 g	146	2 oz	146
Bran Flakes	100 g	318	1 oz	89
avg portion	56 g	178	2 oz	178
Cornflakes	100 g		360	1 oz
avg portion	56 g	202	2 oz	202
Grape Nuts	100 g	366	1 oz	102
avg portion	30 g	110		
Porridge Oats	100 g	368	1 oz	103
avg portion with				
skimmed milk	30 g, raw wt	181	1 oz	181
Shredded Wheat	100 g	325	1 oz	91
avg portion	56 g	182	2 oz	182
Shreddies	100 g	331	1 oz	93
avg portion	56 g	186	2 oz	186
Special K	100 g	377	1 oz	105

Food Groups	Amount	Calories	Amount	Calories
Special K, avg portion	42 g	168	1½ oz	168
Sultana Bran	100 g	303	1 oz	85
avg portion	56 g	170	2 oz	170
Weetabix	100 g	352	1 oz	98
	per biscuit	70		
Wholewheat muesli	100 g	349	1 oz	98
avg portion,				
unsweetened	56 g	196	2 oz	196

DAIRY PRODUCE

Food Groups	Amount	Calories	Amount	Calories
Butter	100 g	737	1 oz	206
	1 tsp	35		
	1 US cup	1648	8 oz	1648
Dairy/fat spread				
blend of cream and oil	100 g	681	1 oz	191
Milk, whole	100 ml	66	1 pint	375
	1 US cup	150	8 fl oz	150
semi - skimmed	100 ml	46	1 pint	261
	1 US cup	105	8 fl oz	105
skimmed	100 ml	33	1 pint	187
	1 US cup	75	8 fl oz	75
condensed, skimmed	100 ml	267	1 fl oz	75
sweetened	1 US cup	600	8 fl oz	600
evaporated	100 ml	151	1 fl oz	42
	1 US cup	336	8 fl oz	336
flavoured,	100 ml	68	1 pint	386

Food Groups	Amount	Calories	Amount	Calories
Milk, flavoured	1 US cup	154	8 fl oz	154
goats	100 ml	60	1 pint	341
	1 US cup	136	8 fl oz	136
soya, plain	100 ml	32	1 pint	182
	1 US cup	73	8 fl oz	73
soya, sweetened with	100 ml	45	1 pint	256
fruit juice	1 US cup	102	8 fl oz	102
Buttermilk	100 ml	41	1 pint	232
	1 US cup	93	8 fl oz	93
Cream, half	100 ml	148	1 fl oz	41
	1 tbsp	22		
	1 US cup	328	8 fl oz	328
single	100 ml	198	1 fl oz	55
	1 tbsp	30		
	1 US cup	440	8 fl oz	440
soured	100 ml	205	1 fl oz	57
	1 tbsp	30		

FOOD GROUPS	AMOUNT	CALORIES	AMOUNT	CALORIES
Cream, soured	1 US cup	456	8 fl oz	456
whipping	100 ml	373	1 fl oz	104
	1 tbsp	56		
	1 US cup	832	8 fl oz	832
double	100 ml	449	1 fl oz	126
	1 tbsp	67		
	1 US cup	1008	8 fl oz	1008
sterilised, tinned	100 ml	239	1 fl oz	67
	1 tbsp	35		
	1 US cup	536	8 fl oz	536
Yogurt, low-fat, natural	100 g	56	1 oz	16
	1 tbsp	10		
	1 US cup	128	8 oz	128
fruit/nut	100 g	90	1 oz	25
	150 g pot	135		
flavoured	100 g	90	1 oz	25
	150 g pot	135		

Food Groups	Amount	Calories	Amount	Calories
Yogurt (cont)				
very-low fat/diet natural	100 g	50	1 oz	14
avg, fruit	100 g	44	1 oz	12
	125g pot	55		
avg, flavoured	100 g	40	1 oz	11
	125 g pot	50		
whole milk, natural	100 g	79	1 oz	22
fruit	100 g	105	1 oz	29
thick & creamy, natural	100 g	110	1 oz	31
fruit	100 g	125	1 oz	35
Greek- style, cows	100 g	130	1 oz	36
Greek- style with honey	100 g	150	1 oz	42
sheep's	100 g	106	1 oz	30
custard-style, fruit, avg	100 g	140	1 oz	39
Drinking yogurt, regular	100 ml	77	1 fl oz	22
low-fat	100 ml	67	1 fl oz	19
Créme fraîche, regular	100 ml	380	1 fl oz	106

FOOD GROUPS	AMOUNT	CALORIES	AMOUNT	CALORIES
Créme fraîche, half-fat	100 ml	169	1 fl oz	47
Fromage frais, plain,				
low-fat	100 g	113	1 oz	32
very-low fat	100 g	58	1 oz	16
fruit/flavoured	100 g	131	1 oz	37
low-fat	100 g	113	1 oz	32
virtually fat-free	100 g	48	1 oz	13
Eggs				
1 egg-boiled/poached	60 g	80	size 3	80
fried	60 g	100	size 3	100
scrambled	60 g	130	size 3	130
yolk only	size 3	65		
white only	size 3	15		
CHEESES				
Austrian smoked cheese	100 g	278	1 oz	78
Brie/Camembert	100 g	308	1 oz	86
Caerphilly	100 g	379	1 oz	106

Food Groups	Amount	Calories	Amount	Calories
Cheddar	100 g	412	1 oz	115
grated	1 US cup	460	4 oz	460
Cheddar-type,				
reduced - fat	100 g	260	1 oz	73
Cheddar - vegetarian	100 g	410	1 oz	115
Cheese spread	100 g	280	1 oz	78
light	100 g	185	1 oz	52
Cheshire	100 g	377	1 oz	105
Cottage cheese,				
plain/chives/pineapple	100 g	100	1 oz	28
half - fat	100 g	86	1 oz	24
Cream cheese	100 g	439	1 oz	123
Danish blue	100 g	347	1 oz	97
Edam/Gouda Cheese	100 g	333	1 oz	93
Full fat soft cheese				
(e.g. Boursin)	100 g	414	1 oz	116
Gruyère	100 g	400	1 oz	112

Food Groups	Amount	Calories	Amount	Calories
Mozzarella	100 g	310	1 oz	87
Parmesan	100 g	388	1 oz	109
grated	1 tbsp	30		
Pizza cheese, grated	100 g	308	1 oz	86
Processed cheese	100 g	330	1 oz	92
Quark (skimmed milk curd cheese)	100 g	70	1 oz	20
Soft cheese, regular (e.g. Philadelphia)	100 g	310	1 oz	87
light	100 g	185	1 oz	52
Stilton/Gorgonzola	100 g	411	1 oz	115
Wensleydale	100 g	375	1 oz	105
Margarine - all types	100 g	739	1 oz	207

NON-DAIRY FATS AND OILS

Food Groups	Amount	Calories	Amount	Calories
Margarine (cont)	1 tsp	35		
low-fat spread	100 g	390	1 oz	109
	1 tsp	15		
very low-fat spread	100 g	265	1 oz	74
	1 tsp	10		
Oil all types	100 ml	899	1 fl oz	252
	1 tbsp	160		
	1 US cup	2016	8 fl oz	2016
French dressing				
(vinaigrette)	100 ml	465	1 fl oz	130
	1 tbsp	84		
	1 US cup	1040	8 fl oz	1040
calorie-reduced,	100 ml	89	1 fl oz	25
	1 tbsp	16		

MEAT AND MEAT PRODUCTS

Food Groups	Amount	Calories	Amount	Calories
BEEF				
Braising steak, lean				
cooked, no added fat	100g serving	170	3½ oz	170
Brisket/salt beef -				
boiled	100 g	326	1 oz	91
Forerib,				
roasted - lean only	100 g	225	1 oz	63
Minced beef, lean				
cooked, drained of fat	100 g	232	1 oz	65
extra lean, cooked	100 g	144	1 oz	40
Steaks, trimmed:				
(lean only) grilled	100 g	168	1 oz	47
avg steak, grilled	140 g	235		
Sirloin, lean only,				
roasted/grilled	100 g	192	1 oz	54

Food Groups	Amount	Calories	Amount	Calories
avg steak, grilled	170 g raw wt	340		
Fillet, avg steak, grilled				
raw weight	170 g	250		
Topside				
roasted, lean only	100 g	156	1 oz	44
Hamburger, lean				
grilled	113 g	240		
low-fat grilled	each	105		
Beef sausages,				
chipolatas - grilled	per sausage	75		
large - grilled	per sausage	150		
PORK AND BACON				
Bacon, lean				
/trimmed- raw	100 g	260	1 oz	73
grilled	per rasher	65		
Ham/Gammon joint, -				
boiled (lean)	100 g	167	1 oz	47

Food Groups	Amount	Calories	Amount	Calories
Gammon steak,				
lean-grilled	170 g	290		
Pork, leg roast				
lean	100 g	185	1 oz	52
loin chop or chump				
steak boneless, trimmed,				
grilled	113 g	255		
fillet, grilled/casseroled	100 g	142	1 oz	40
spare rib chop,				
trimmed of fat	per chop	275	4 oz	275
Chinese spare rib,	per rib	230	3 oz	230
Chipolatas pork sausages				
grilled	per sausage	90		
large grilled	per sausage	180		
low-fat grilled	per sausage	85		
cocktail	per sausage	45		

Food Groups	Amount	Calories	Amount	Calories
LAMB				
Lamb leg roast, lean	100 g	191	1 oz	53
shoulder roast, lean	100 g	196	1 oz	55
loin chop/cutlet,				
bone in,	per chop	205		
neck fillet,	100 g	232	1 oz	65
VEAL				
Fillet/escalope -				
roast	100 g	230	1 oz	65
grilled with egg				
and breadcrumbs	100 g	215	1 oz	60
OFFAL				
Kidney, all types				
fried	100 g	155	1 oz	43
Liver, calves				
fried	100 g	254	1 oz	71
lamb's, fried	100 g	232	1 oz	65

FOOD GROUPS	AMOUNT	CALORIES	AMOUNT	CALORIES
Liver, chicken				
fried	100 g	194	1 oz	54
Oxtail, stewed, lean only	100 g	243	1 oz	68
Sweetbreads, lamb				
crumbed and fried	100 g	230	1 oz	65
DELICATESSEN				
Black pudding,				
sliced and fried	100 g	304	1 oz	85
Corned beef	100 g	205	1 oz	57
	per slice	80		
Cornish pastie	small	395		
	large	550		
Danish salami	100 g	535	1 oz	150
	per slice	60		
Frankfurters	100 g	335	1 oz	94
	per sausage	235		

Food Groups	Amount	Calories	Amount	Calories
Garlic sausage	100 g	135	1 oz	38
	per slice	15		
German salami	100 g	418	1 oz	117
	per slice	42		
Ham, lean	100 g	150	1 oz	42
	per slice	40		
Liver sausage	100 g	238	1 oz	67
	per slice	25		
	per slice	14		
Pastrami	100g	120	1 oz	34
	per slice	15		
Pâté, liver,	100 g	316	1 oz	88
reduced fat	100 g	191	1 oz	53
Pork pie, small	each	270		
Sausage roll,	56 g each	202		
Scotch egg	per egg	280		
Tongue	100 g	179	1 oz	50

POULTRY AND GAME

Food Groups	Amount	Calories	Amount	Calories
Turkey breast	100 g	100	1 oz	28
Chicken meat				
roast (no skin)	100 g	148	1 oz	41
breast portion skinned,				
on the bone, grilled	170 g	145		
drumstick, skinned and				
grilled,	100 g	65		
Duck, meat only -				
roast	100 g	189	1 oz	53
Goose, meat only, roast	100 g	319	1 oz	89
Pheasant,				
meat only - roast	100 g	213	1 oz	60
Rabbit, meat only -				
casseroled	100 g	179	1 oz	50
Turkey, meat only -				
roast	100 g	140	1 oz	39

Food Groups	Amount	Calories	Amount	Calories
Turkey sausage, grilled	per sausage	165		
Venison,				
roast	100 g	198	1 oz	55

FISH AND FISH PRODUCTS

Food Groups	Amount	Calories	Amount	Calories
Anchovies,				
tinned, drained	100 g	280	1 oz	78
per fillet	each	10		
Bass, fillet,				
steamed, avg portion	140 g	175	5 oz	175
Clams, tinned	100 g	107	1 oz	30
Cod, fillet,				
crumbed, baked	100 g	190	1 oz	53
crumbed, avg portion	140 g	266	5 oz	266
steamed/baked				
avg portion	140 g	134	5 oz	134
Crab, cooked/dressed	100 g	127	1 oz	35
Haddock,				
fillet crumbed, baked	100 g	192	1 oz	54
avg portion	140 g	270	5 oz	270
steamed/baked	100 g	98	1 oz	27

Food Groups	Amount	Calories	Amount	Calories
avg portion	140 g	137	5 oz	
Smoked haddock,				
steamed	100 g	101	1 oz	28
avg portion	140 g	141	5 oz	141
Herring fillet,				
grilled	100 g	199	1 oz	56
whole herring, grilled	140 g	190	5 oz	190
Rollmops	100 g	230	1 oz	64
each	56 g	128	2 oz	128
Kipper fillet,				
baked/steamed	100 g	205	1 oz	57
avg portion	84 g	180	3 oz	180
Mackerel fillet,				
smoked	100 g	360	1 oz	100
avg smoked fillet	98 g	353	3½ oz	353
Plaice,				

Food Groups	Amount	Calories	Amount	Calories
steamed fillet	100 g	93	1 oz	26
avg portion	113 g	105	4 oz	105
crumbed, fried	100 g	228	1 oz	64
avg portion	113 g	258	4 oz	258
Prawns, cooked				
and shelled	100 g	107	1 oz	30
Salmon, grilled				
baked steak (boned)	252 g	302	9 oz	302
tinned	100 g	155	1 oz	43
Smoked salmon	100 g	142	1 oz	40
Sardines, fresh				
whole sardine, grilled	50 g	98		
tinned in tomato sauce	100 g	177	1 oz	50
Sole				
whole fish, steamed	213 g	194	7½ oz	194
crumbed fillet	100 g	195	1 oz	55
Trout,whole				

FOOD GROUPS	AMOUNT	CALORIES	AMOUNT	CALORIES
Trout grilled/baked	283 g	250	10 oz	250
Tuna,				
in oil, drained	100 g	189	1 oz	53
in brine, drained	100 g	99	1 oz	28
Fish fingers, grilled	per finger	50		
Fish cake crumbed, grilled	per cake	80		

VEGETARIAN

Food Groups	Amount	Calories	Amount	Calories
Quorn	100 g	86	1 oz	24
Tofu, plain	100 g	90	1 oz	25
marinated	100 g	208	1 oz	58
Sausages, grilled	per sausage	60		
Burgers / cutlets	per item	135		

FRUIT

Calories for raw, fresh fruit have been calculated including
skin, pips, stones etc

Food Groups	Amount	Calories	Amount	Calories
Apples, eating	100 g	42	1 oz	12
avg whole fruit	113 g	48	4 oz	113
cooking	100 g	26	1 oz	7
avg whole fruit	227 g	56	8 oz	56
apple sauce, sweetened	1 tbsp	20		
unsweetened	1 tbsp	10		
Apricots, fresh	100 g	29	1 oz	8
avg whole fruit	28 g	8	8 oz	8
dried (without stones)	100 g	158	1 oz	44
per dried fruit		10		
tinned in juice	100 g	34	1 oz	10
Avocado	100 g	134	1 oz	38
avg half fruit/				
Hass variety		125		
Bananas	100 g	62	1 oz	17

FOOD GROUPS	AMOUNT	CALORIES	AMOUNT	CALORIES
avg medium fruit	142 g	85	5 oz	85
Blackberries, raw/frozen	100 g	25	1 oz	7
stewed with sugar	100 g	56	1 oz	16
Blackcurrants, raw/frozen	100 g	28	1 oz	8
Blueberries, raw/frozen	100 g	64	1 oz	18
Cherries, raw	100 g	39	1 oz	11
glacé	100 g	251	1 oz	70
	1 US cup	490	7 oz	490
per glacé/cocktail cherry		10		
Cranberries, raw/frozen	100 g	14	1 oz	4
Clementines, satsumas,				
tangerines	100 g	28	1 oz	8
per medium fruit	100 g	28	3½ oz	28
Currants	100 g	267	1 oz	76
	1 US cup	380	5 oz	380
Dates, dried with stones	100 g	227	1 oz	64
dried, stoned	100 g	290	1 oz	81

Food Groups	Amount	Calories	Amount	Calories
per dried date		15		
Dried fruit salad	100 g	185	1 oz	52
Figs, fresh	100 g	43	1 oz	12
per fresh fruit		15		
dried	100 g	227	1 oz	64
per dried fruit		30		
Fruit cocktail,				
tinned in juice	100 g	29	1 oz	8
Gooseberries, raw	100 g	19	1 oz	5
stewed with sugar	100 g	54	1 oz	15
Grapefruit, fresh	100 g	20	1 oz	6
avg medium fruit		50		
tinned in juice	100 g	30	1 oz	8
Grapes	100 g	57	1 oz	16
Kiwi fruit	100 g	42	1 oz	12
avg whole fruit	each	35		
Lemon	100 g	19	1 oz	5

Food Groups	Amount	Calories	Amount	Calories
Lychees, raw	100 g	36	1 oz	10
tinned in syrup	100 g	68	1 oz	19
Mandarins,				
tinned in juice	100 g	32	1 oz	9
Melon, honeydew	100 g	19	1 oz	5
avg slice	226 g	40	8 oz	40
Olives, with stones	100 g	82	1 oz	23
per black olive	each	3		
per stuffed olive	each	5		
Oranges	100 g	26		7
avg whole fruit	255 g	63	9 oz	63
Passion fruit	100 g	22	1 oz	6
avg whole fruit	50 g	11		
Peaches, fresh	100 g	30	1 oz	8
avg whole fruit	170 g	48	6 oz	48
tinned in juice	100 g	39	1 oz	11
Pears, fresh	100 g	36	1 oz	10

Food Groups	Amount	Calories	Amount	Calories
avg whole fruit	170 g	60	6 oz	60
tinned in juice	100 g	33	1 oz	9
Pineapple fresh, flesh	100 g	41	1 oz	11
avg slice	140 g	35	5 oz	35
tinned in juice	100 g	47	1 oz	13
Plums, fresh	100 g	34	1 oz	10
avg whole fruit	70 g	24		
stewed with sugar	100 g	75	1 oz	21
Prunes, ready-to-eat	100 g	141	1 oz	40
tinned in juice	100 g	79	1 oz	22
per prune	each	10		
Raisins/sultanas	100 g	272	1 oz	76
	1 US cup	456	6 oz	456
Raspberries/				
Strawberries, fresh	100 g	25	1 oz	7
Rhubarb, raw	100 g	7	1 oz	2
stewed with sugar	100 g	48	1 oz	14

VEGETABLES

Calories for raw vegetables have been calculated from
their prepared weight, ie peeled, stems trimmed, outer
leaves removed.

FOOD GROUPS	AMOUNT	CALORIES	AMOUNT	CALORIES
Asparagus, raw/steamed	100 g	26	1 oz	7
per spear	each	7		
Aubergine, raw	100 g	15	1 oz	4
avg whole aubergine	198 g	30	7 oz	30
Bamboo shoots, tinned	100 g	7	1 oz	2
Beans -				
Baked beans,				
tinned in tomato sauce	100 g	84	1 oz	24
Baked beans tinned				
with reduced sugar	100 g	73	1 oz	21
Butter beans, dried	100 g	275	1 oz	75
cooked/tinned	100 g	77	1 oz	22
Cannelini beans,				
tinned	100 g	85	1 oz	24
Kidney beans, raw	100 g	266	1 oz	75

Food Groups	Amount	Calories	Amount	Calories
cooked/tinned	100 g	100	1 oz	28
Broad beans, raw	100 g	121	1 oz	34
cooked	100 g	107	1 oz	30
Chick peas, dried	100 g	320	1 oz	91
cooked/tinned	100 g	115	1 oz	32
Green beans,				
runner/French	100 g	24	1 oz	7
Soya beans, tinned	100 g	140	1 oz	39
Mixed Bean Salad,				
tinned	100 g	90	1 oz	25
Beansprouts, raw/boiled	100 g	31	1 oz	9
stir-fried	100 g	72	1 oz	20
Beetroot, boiled	100 g	46	1 oz	13
Broccoli, raw	100 g	33	1 oz	9
steamed,boiled	100 g	24	1 oz	7
Brussels sprouts, raw	100 g	42	1 oz	12
steamed/boiled	100 g	35	1 oz	10

FOOD GROUPS	AMOUNT	CALORIES	AMOUNT	CALORIES
Cabbage, raw	100 g	26	1 oz	7
steamed/boiled	100 g	16	1 oz	5
Coleslaw, in mayonnaise	100 g	167	1 oz	47
reduced-calorie dressing	100 g	95	1 oz	27
Carrots, raw, peeled	100 g	35	1 oz	10
boiled	100 g	24	1 oz	7
per avg carrot	each	15		
Cauliflower, raw,				
florets only	100 g	34	1 oz	10
boiled	100 g	28	1 oz	8
Celeriac, raw	100 g	28	1 oz	8
boiled	100 g	14	1 oz	4
Celery, raw/boiled	100 g	7	1 oz	2
per stick		5		
Corn on the cob,				
whole cob boiled	198 g	117	7 oz	117
Courgette/zucchini,				

Food Groups	Amount	Calories	Amount	Calories
raw/boiled	100 g	18	1 oz	5
stir-fried	100 g	63	1 oz	18
Cucumber, raw	100 g	10	1 oz	3
Fennel, raw/boiled	100 g	12	1 oz	4
Gherkins, pickled	100 g	14	1 oz	4
Leeks, raw/boiled	100 g	22	1 oz	6
Lentils, red split, raw	100 g	318	1 oz	89
cooked	100 g	100	1 oz	28
Lettuce, raw	100 g	14	1 oz	4
Mange-tout peas, raw	100 g	32	1 oz	9
boiled	100 g	26	1 oz	7
stir-fried	100 g	71	1 oz	20
Mixed vegetables, (frozen) boiled	100 g	42	1 oz	12
Marrow, raw/boiled	100 g	12	1 oz	3
Mushrooms, raw/tinned	100 g	13	1 oz	4
stir-fried with butter	100 g	157	1 oz	44

FOOD GROUPS	AMOUNT	CALORIES	AMOUNT	CALORIES
in garlic breadcrumbs	each	35		
Onions, raw	100 g	36	1 oz	10
fried	100 g	164	1 oz	46
pickled onion	each	5		
cocktail onion	each	1		
spring onion	each	3		
Parsnips, raw, peeled	100 g	66	1 oz	18
roast	100 g	107	1 oz	30
Peas, fresh, raw	100 g	68	1 oz	19
frozen, raw	100 g	54	1 oz	15
tinned, garden	100 g	46	1 oz	13
tinned, processed	100 g	82	1 oz	23
Peppers, raw	100 g	15	1 oz	4
avg whole pepper	each	15		
Potatoes, avg,				
raw, peeled	100 g	70	1 oz	20
small baked with skin	198 g	150	7 oz	150

Food Groups	Amount	Calories	Amount	Calories
large baked with skin	350 g	245	12½ oz	245
mashed with butter	100 g	104	1 oz	29
roast/sauté	100 g	149	1 oz	42
avg medium roast	56 g	84	2 oz	84
French Fries	100 g	280	1 oz	78
thick cut chips	100 g	189	1 oz	53
Oven chips, baked	100 g	162	1 oz	45
croquette potato, baked	each	50		
hash browns, baked	each	80		
Pumpkin, raw, flesh only	100 g	13	1 oz	4
Radish	each	2		
Ratatouille	100 g	55	1 oz	15
Red Cabbage				
with apple, cooked	100 g	122	1 oz	34
Spinach, raw,				
stems removed	100 g	25	1 oz	7
steamed	100 g	19	1 oz	5

FOOD GROUPS	AMOUNT	CALORIES	AMOUNT	CALORIES
Spring greens, raw,				
stems removed	100 g	33	1 oz	9
steamed	100 g	20	1 oz	6
Sweetcorn, kernels,				
tinned	100 g	85	1 oz	24
Whole baby sweetcorn	100 g	36	1 oz	10
Tomatoes, fresh/tinned	100 g	17	1 oz	5
Turnips, raw, peeled	100 g	23	1 oz	7
boiled	100 g	12	1 oz	3
Watercress, raw	100 g	22	1 oz	6

NUTS AND SEEDS

Food Groups	Amount	Calories	Amount	Calories
Almonds, shelled	100 g	612	1 oz	171
	per whole nut	10		
Brazil nuts, shelled	100 g	682	1 oz	191
	per whole nut	20		
Cashew Nuts, shelled	100 g	611	1 oz	171
	per whole nut	15		
Chestnuts, shelled	100 g	170	1 oz	48
Coconut, fresh	100 g	357	1 oz	100
desiccated	100 g	604	1 oz	169
	1 US cup	302		
creamed	100g	669	1 oz	187
Hazelnuts, shelled	100 g	650	1 oz	182
	per whole nut	8		
Mixed nuts, chopped	100 g	607	1 oz	170
	1 US cup	698	4 oz	698
Peanuts, plain, shelled	100 g	564	1 oz	158

Food Groups	Amount	Calories	Amount	Calories
roasted, salted	100 g	602	1 oz	169
	per whole nut	5		
Pecan nuts	100 g	688	1 oz	193
	per whole nut	15		
Pine nuts	100 g	688	1 oz	193
Pistachio nuts, shelled	100 g	643	1 oz	180
Sesame seeds	100 g	598	1 oz	170
Sunflower seeds	100 g	581	1 oz	163
Walnuts	100 g	688	1 oz	193
chopped	1 US cup	772	4 oz	772
per walnut half	each	15		

CAKES, BISCUITS AND CRISPS

These are only average figures. There is a good deal of
variation between different manufacturers and different
recipes. Nutritional information is generally given on pack-
aged items so check the panel for an accurate calorie value.

Food Groups	Amount	Calories	Amount	Calories
CAKES				
Chelsea Bun	each	190		
Cherry Cake	per slice	200		
Chocolate Brownie	each	300		
Crumpet, toasted	each	80		
with butter	each	120		
Currant bun	each	179		
Custard tart	each	230		
Danish pastry	each	360		
Doughnut, sugared ring	each	240		
jam	each	304		
Eclair, chocolate				
iced and cream filled	each	155		
Fruit cake, light	per slice	220		

Food Groups	Amount	Calories	Amount	Calories
rich/Christmas cake	per slice	305		
Gingerbread	per slice	178		
Greek baklava	each	322		
Hot cross bun, toasted	each	175		
with butter	each	215		
wholemeal	each	195		
Jam tart	each	140		
Macaroon	each	145		
Madeira cake	average slice	140		
Malt loaf	average slice	110		
Mince pie	each	235		
Muffin, plain	each	140		
chocolate chip	each	170		
Scone, plain	each	183		
currant	each	195		
cheese	each	250		
Scotch pancake	each	85		

Food Groups	Amount	Calories	Amount	Calories
Waffle	each	165		
with 1 tbsp syrup	each	255		
BISCUITS				
Bourbon	each	60		
Cereal bar (avg)	each	125		
Cheese straw	each	15		
Chocolate Chip	each	55		
Chocolate digestive	each	85		
Cream cracker	each	35		
Crispbread, average	each	25		
Custard cream	each	60		
Digestive	each	70		
Fig roll	each	65		
Flapjack	per slice	120		
French toast	each	30		
Garibaldi	each	35		
Gingernut	each	50		

FOOD GROUPS	AMOUNT	CALORIES	AMOUNT	CALORIES
Grissini	each	20		
Marie	each	25		
Matzos	each	70		
Melba toast	each	15		
Nice	each	45		
Rice cake	each	25		
Rich tea	each	40		
Shortbread (chunky)	each	110		
Petticoat tail	each	65		
Water biscuit	each	25		
Wholemeal bran biscuit	each	65		
Crisps, plain	25 g	120	1 oz bag	120
flavoured	25 g	135	1 oz bag	135
reduced - fat	25 g	120	1 oz bag	120
Bombay mix	100 g	490	1 oz	137
Tortilla chips	100 g	480	1 oz	135

PRESERVES AND CONDIMENTS

Food Groups	Amount	Calories	Amount	Calories
SWEET				
Chocolate spread	100 g	304	1 oz	85
Hazelnut Chocolate				
spread	100 g	549	1 oz	154
	1 teaspoon	55		
Honey	100 g	288	1 oz	81
	1 teaspoon	40		
	1 US cup	972	12 oz	972
Jam, regular	100 g	261	1 oz	73
	1 teaspoon	35		
reduced - sugar	100 g	123	1 oz	35
	1 teaspoon	17		
Lemon curd	100 g	283	1 oz	79
	1 teaspoon	40		
Marmalade	100 g	261	1 oz	73
	1 teaspoon	35		

FOOD GROUPS	AMOUNT	CALORIES	AMOUNT	CALORIES
Marmalade				
reduced - sugar	100 g	135	1 oz	38
	1 teaspoon	17		
Mincemeat	100 g	274	1 oz	77
	1 tbsp	95		
Peanut butter	100 g	623	1 oz	175
	1 teaspoon	60		
	1 US cup	1400	8 oz	1400
Sugar	100 g	394	1 oz	110
	1 teaspoon	20		
	1 US cup	770	7 oz	770
Syrup	100 g	298	1 oz	83
	1 tbsp	90		
	1 US cup	1400	8 oz	1400
Treacle	100 g	257	1 oz	72
	1 tbsp	77		
	1 US cup	828	11 ½ oz	828

FOOD GROUPS	AMOUNT	CALORIES	AMOUNT	CALORIES
SAVOURY				
Apple sauce	100 g	74	1 oz	21
	1 tbsp	20		
Blue cheese dressing	1 tbsp	45		
Bread sauce	100 g	110	1 oz	31
	1 tbsp	20		
Cranberry sauce	100 g	232	1 oz	65
	1 teaspoon	35		
Horseradish	1 teaspoon	10		
Mango chutney	100 g	285	1 oz	80
	1 tbsp	85		
Mayonnaise, traditional	100 g	691	1 oz	193
	1 tbsp	150		
reduced - calorie	100 g	286	1 oz	80
	1 tbsp	44		
Mint sauce	1 teaspoon	2		
Mustard	1 teaspoon	10		

Food Groups	Amount	Calories	Amount	Calories
Pickle	100 g	134	1 oz	38
	1 tbsp	40		
Redcurrant jelly	100 g	273	1 oz	76
	1 teaspoon	40		
Relish, barbecue	1 tbsp	30		
corn	1 tbsp	30		
Salad cream, regular	100 g	348	1 oz	98
	1 tbsp	50		
reduced - calorie	100 g	194	1 oz	54
	1 tbsp	25		
Soy sauce	1 tbsp	13		
Tomato ketchup	100 g	98	1 oz	27
	1 tbsp	20		
Tomato puree	100 g	68	1 oz	19
	1 tbsp	13		
Yeast extract	100 g	172	1 oz	48
	1 teaspoon	26		

SWEETS AND CHOCOLATES

Food Groups	Amount	Calories	Amount	Calories
Barley sugar	each	25		
Butter toffee popcorn	100 g	400	1 oz	112
Butterscotch	each	25		
Chocolate,				
milk or plain	100 g	536	1 oz	150
Chocolates,				
mixed selection	100 g	465	1 oz	130
Chocolate-covered				
brazil nut	each	55		
Chocolate with mint				
cream centre	each	35		
Chocolate truffle	each	60		
Coconut ice	100 g	392	1 oz	110
Fruit pastilles	each	17		
Fudge	100 g	568	1 oz	160
Marshmallow	each	20		

Food Groups	Amount	Calories	Amount	Calories
Marzipan	100 g	404	1 oz	113
Mint/boiled sweet	each	30		
Nougat	100 g	375	1 oz	105
Sugared almonds	each	15		
Toffees	each	35		
Turkish Delight	100 g	295	1 oz	83
chocolate covered	100 g	365	1 oz	102
Popular Chocolate Bars				
Aero - snack size	each	120		
Blue Riband	each	105		
Bounty - fun size	each	135		
Cadbury's Creme Egg	each	175		
Crunchie - small bar	each	110		
treat size	each	80		
Double Decker, treat size	each	85		
Flake - treat size	each	75		
Fudge - treat size	each	65		

Food Groups	Amount	Calories	Amount	Calories
Galaxy - small bar	each	245		
Kit Kat - 2 finger bar	each	108		
Lion Bar - mini	each	80		
Maltesers - fun size	per packet	105		
M & M's - fun size	per packet	125		
Marathon - fun size	each	90		
Mars Bar - snack size	each	180		
Milky Bar - small	12.6 g	65		
Milky Way - fun size	each	75		
Rolos	per chocolate	25		
Smarties, fun pack	per pack	55		
Time Out - treat size	each	105		
Toffee Crisp - mini	each	88		
Twirl - treat size	each	115		
Twix	per bar	140		
Wispa - treat size	each	80		

BEVERAGES

Food Groups	Amount	Calories	Amount	Calories
SOFT DRINKS				
Juices, unsweetened				
Apple	100 ml	38	1 fl oz	11
Blackcurrant	100 ml	60	1 fl oz	17
Cranberry	100 ml	49	1 fl oz	14
Grape	100 ml	46	1 fl oz	13
Grapefruit	100 ml	33	1 fl oz	9
Orange	100 ml	36	1 fl oz	10
Pineapple	100 ml	41	1 fl oz	11
Tomato	100 ml	14	1 fl oz	4
Hot chocolate or				
malted drink	100 ml	90	1 fl oz	25
made with whole milk				
avg serving	227 ml	200	8 fl oz	200
made with skimmed milk				
avg serving	227 ml	160	8 fl oz	160

Food Groups	Amount	Calories	Amount	Calories
Milk shakes, avg	100 ml	87	1 fl oz	24
made with				
whole milk	284 ml	245	½ pt	245
	avg serving			
Milk shake made with				
semi- skimmed milk	100 ml	69	1 fl oz	20
	284 ml	200	½ pt	200
	avg serving			
American Ginger Ale	100 ml	39	1 fl oz	11
Bitter lemon	100 ml	35	1 fl oz	10
Cola	100 ml	39	1 fl oz	11
Dry Ginger	100 ml	18	1 fl oz	5
Lemonade	100 ml	25	1 fl oz	7
Tonic Water	100 ml	25	1 fl oz	7

ALCOHOLIC DRINKS

Food Groups	Amount	Calories	Amount	Calories
SPIRITS				
25 ml/⅙ gill (standard				
pub measure)				
Brandy, Gin, Rum,				
Tequila, Vodka	25 ml	50		
Whisky, Scotch, Bourbon	25 ml	50		
Campari	25 ml	55		
Ouzo/Pernod	25 ml	65		
Southern Comfort	25 ml	70		
Jack Daniels	25 ml	60		
Aperitifs				
50 ml/⅓ gill				
standard pub measure				
Sherry - dry	50 ml	58		
medium	50 ml	59		
sweet	50 ml	68		

Food Groups	Amount	Calories	Amount	Calories
Cinzano extra dry	50 ml	50		
Cinzano Rose	50 ml	70		
Dubonnet dry	50 ml	55		
Dubonnet red	50 ml	75		
Martini Bianco/Rosso	50 ml	90		
Martini Rose	50 ml	85		
COCKTAILS				
(These tend to be double measures)				
Gin and tonic	50 ml spirit	145		
Pimm's with lemonade	50 ml alcohol	140		
Snowball - Advocaat and lemonade	50 ml alcohol	170		
Pina Colada	50 ml alcohol	170		
Tequila Sunrise	50 ml spirit	165		
Harvey Wallbanger	50 ml spirit	160		
Whisky and dry ginger	50 ml spirit	180		

FOOD GROUPS	AMOUNT	CALORIES	AMOUNT	CALORIES
Rum and Coke	50 ml spirit	175		
Dubonnet & lemonade	50 ml alcohol	110		
White wine spritzer	250 ml	115		
WINES per avg glass 142 ml/5 fl oz				
Red	142 ml	96		
Rose	142 ml	100		
White - dry	142 ml	94		
medium	142 ml	105		
sparkling	142 ml	105		
sweet	142 ml	133		
Champagne	142 ml	105		
BEERS AND LAGERS				
284 ml/½ pint glass				
Beer, draught	284 ml	90	½ pint	
Guinness	284 ml	90	½ pint	
lager, bottled	284 ml	80	½ pint	

Food Groups	Amount	Calories	Amount	Calories
low alcohol	284 ml	56	½ pint	
Pale Ale	284 ml	90	½ pint	
Stout	284 ml	105	½ pint	
Cider - dry	284 ml	102	½ pint	
sweet	284 ml	119	½ pint	
vintage	284 ml	285	½ pint	
LIQUEURS				
per 25 ml/⅛ gill measure				
Armagnac	25 ml	60		
Calvados	25 ml	60		
Grand Marnier	25 ml	80		
Tia Maria	25 ml	75		
Cointreau/Drambuie	25 ml	85		

POPULAR DISHES

Starters

All calories are based on average portion sizes.
However they can only serve as a rough guide as recipes
vary enormously.

Food Groups	Amount	Calories	Amount	Calories
½ Avocado with 1 tbsp vinaigrette dressing		210		
Asparagus spears with 1 tbsp mayonnaise,		205		
Humus with pitta bread		275		
with raw vegetable crudités		145		
Melon		40		
Melon with parma ham		150		
Pate with melba toast (no butter)		220		
Prawn Cocktail		200		
Soups - cream of chicken / mushroom	284 ml	156	½ pint	156

Food Groups	Amount	Calories	Amount	Calories
cream of tomato	284 ml	190	½ pint	190
celery	284 ml	95	½ pint	95
clam chowder	284 ml	255	½ pint	255
French onion	284 ml	77	½ pint	77
with cheese croûte		250		
gazpacho	284 ml	85	½ pint	
leek and potato	284 ml	110	½ pint	110
lentil	284 ml	280	½ pint	280
minestrone	284 ml	75	½ pint	75
oxtail	284 ml	125	½ pint	125
pea and ham	284 ml	130	½ pint	130
tomato	284 ml	88	½ pint	88
vegetable	284 ml	105	½ pint	105
watercress	284 ml	147	½ pint	147
Tabouleh (cracked wheat salad)	per portion	150		
Taramaslata with				

FOOD GROUPS	AMOUNT	CALORIES	AMOUNT	CALORIES
pitta bread		440		
Tzatziki - with raw				
vegetable crudités		85		
with pitta bread		250		
MAIN COURSES **Ready prepared meals**				
British				
Omelette - plain	2 eggs	210		
with 28 g/1 oz cheese		330		
Baked jacket potato				
(350 g/12 ½ oz)				
with 113 g/4 oz				
baked beans		340		
Beef Casserole,				
lean beef		330		
Cauliflower Cheese				
(main course portion)		280		

Food Groups	Amount	Calories	Amount	Calories
Chicken Kiev		345		
Fish Pie, with mashed				
potato topping		310		
Kedgeree		375		
Lancashire hot pot		380		
Macaroni cheese		530		
Meat loaf		265		
Nut roast		330		
Peppered steak				
with mushrooms		345		
Quiche, cheese		385		
Roast beef (lean) with				
Yorkshire pudding				
and gravy		370		
Roast turkey with				
bacon roll, stuffing				
and gravy		310		

FOOD GROUPS	AMOUNT	CALORIES	AMOUNT	CALORIES
Scampi		315		
Shepherds pie		325		
Vegetable cottage pie		250		
Steak and Kidney pie		420		
Indian				
Beef curry		310		
with rice		460		
Chicken tikka		225		
Chicken tikka masala		400		
Lamb biryani		495		
Prawn curry with rice		400		
Tandoori chicken,				
per skinned portion		165		
Lentil dhal		240		
Mixed vegetable curry		145		
Mushroom dopiaza		150		
Onion bhajii (small)	each	85		

Food Groups	Amount	Calories	Amount	Calories
Pilau rice	per portion	225		
Raita - cucumber	1 tbsp	20		
Samosas, small				
meat filled	each	120		
vegetable filled	each	110		
Italian				
Garlic bread	¼ baguette	160		
Canneloni/Lasagne		525		
Pizza - margherita		570		
four seasons		690		
mushroom		555		
pepperoni		725		
Risotto, shellfish		470		
Spaghetti bolognese		536		
Bolognese sauce only		245		
Greek				
Dolmas with salad	each	80		

Food Groups	Amount	Calories	Amount	Calories
Moussaka		415		
Shish kebab		320		
McDonalds				
Hamburger		250		
Cheeseburger		300		
Big Mac		550		
French fries, regular		290		
Chinese				
Barbecue spare ribs	each	140		
Beef with ginger				
and spring onion		295		
Chicken Chow Mein				
(with noodles)		415		
Chicken satay		245		
Crispy aromatic duck				
(1 filled pancake)		145		
Egg fried rice		295		

Food Groups	Amount	Calories	Amount	Calories
Lemon chicken		295		
Prawn chop suey		310		
Sweet and sour pork		195		
Mexican				
Chilli con carne		340		
with brown rice		518		
Guacamole				
(avocado dip)	100 g	275	1 oz	77
1 Tortilla pancake				
(enchilada) filled		290		
PUDDINGS AND DESSERTS				
All calories per portion				
Bakewell Tart		335		
Bread & Butter Pudding		330		
Cheesecake, New York Deli				
- style (lemon, sultana)		155		

FOOD GROUPS	AMOUNT	CALORIES	AMOUNT	CALORIES
with fruit topping		230		
low-fat		204		
Chocolate fudge cake		310		
Christmas pudding		300		
Crème caramel		150		
Crème brûlée		285		
Custard, made with				
whole milk	568ml	570	1 pint	570
custard made with				
semi-skimmed milk	568 ml	450	1 pint	450
Fruit crumble		425		
Fruit salad		130		
Gâteau, with fresh cream		250		
Ice Cream, Cornish vanilla	56 g	110	2 oz	
chocolate (luxury style)	56 g	118	2 oz	
non-dairy vanilla	56 g	95	2 oz	